ESSENTIAL OILS
15 Celebrity Face
& Body Recipes

DIY Luxury Rich & Famous Skin Care Products For Everyone

by Katherine Townsend

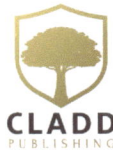

CLADD
PUBLISHING

Cladd Publishing Inc.
USA

This publication is designed to provide accurate information regarding the subject matter covered. It is sold with the understanding that neither the author nor the publisher is providing medical, legal or other professional advice or services. Always seek advice from a competent professional before using any of the information in this book. The author and the publisher specifically disclaim any liability that is incurred from the use or application of the contents of this book.

Essential Oils 15 Celebrity Face & Body Recipes: DIY Luxury Rich & Famous Skin Care Products For Everyone

ISBN 978-1-946881-34-2 (e-book)
ISBN 978-1-946881-33-5 (paperback)

Contents

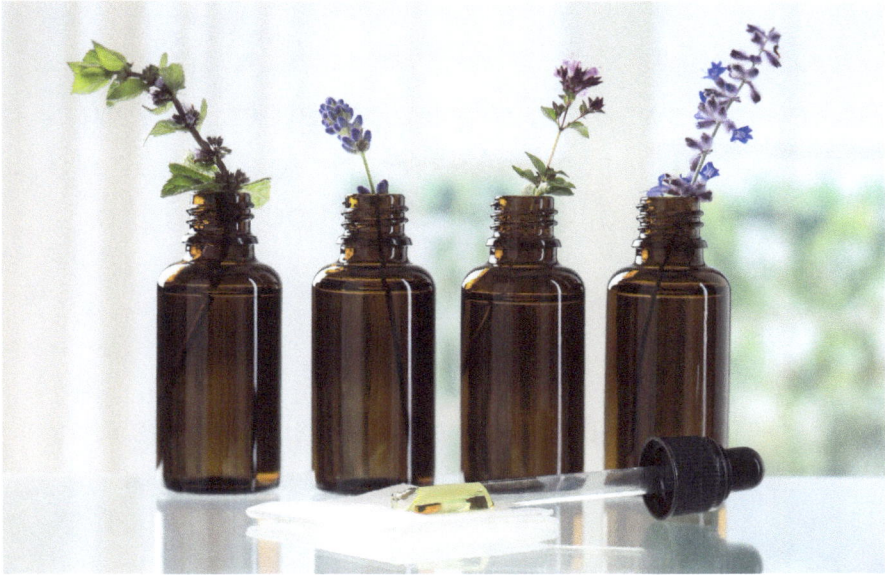

Commonly Asked Questions

Q: CAN I DO THESE RECIPES WITH LITTLE EXPERIENCE AND ON A BUDGET?

A: Yes, while the recipes are based on luxurious products they are budget friendly, non-toxic formulas. This is an excellent book for normal people wanting to enhance their life with high priced essential oil products; but do not want to purchase the expensive version from a specialty store.

Q: WHAT DOES EO MEAN?

A: EO or EOs is the abbreviation for Essential Oils. It is commonly used and will be used in this book.

Q: CAN I SUBSTITUTE ESSENTIAL OILS?

A: You can swap out oils or substitute for your favorite in almost all cases. However, do not use citrus essential oils for products you intend to wear directly in the sun.

Q: GLASS BOTTLE OR PLASTIC?

A: Essential oils can degrade plastic. That is why its recommended to store oils in glass.

Q: BASE PRODUCT VS. CARRIER OIL?

A: A base product is a cream, lotion, shampoo, gel or anything that has already been made. You can add a few drops of essential oils to enhance the product. A carrier oil is a pure oil, that is used to dilute the strength of EOs, and help prolong its aroma.

As a rule of thumb, I wouldn't apply essential oils directly onto your skin without diluting it in a carrier oil first. Although, there are some that you can do this with, unless you are experienced avoid direct application.

Q: CAN I ADJUST THE STRENGTH OF THE RECIPE?

A: Yes, you can and should limit the drops of essential oils based on your personal sensitivity towards the strength. Most recipes in this book are medium strength. However, you can always reduce or increase slightly in either direction unless stated.

FRAGRANCE OIL VS. PURE 100% ESSENTIAL OIL

A: 100% pure essential oils are required for these incredible recipes. Do not purchase "fragrance oil" or "perfume oil" as these can be synthetic and don't provide the desired health benefits. Instead, look for oils that say, "pure essential oil" or "100% essential oil" for the highest quality.

Essential oils come from plants, while fragrance oils are usually artificially created and will contain synthetic chemicals. Even though they smell similar and cost less, they do not provide the same therapeutic benefits.

Q: RAW, ORGANIC AND NATURAL

A: For the highest quality ingredients use raw and or cold pressed honey, coconut, shea butter, aloe vera, jojoba, beeswax, cocoa, and sweet almond oil. Try your best to obtain supplies that are organic and or natural.

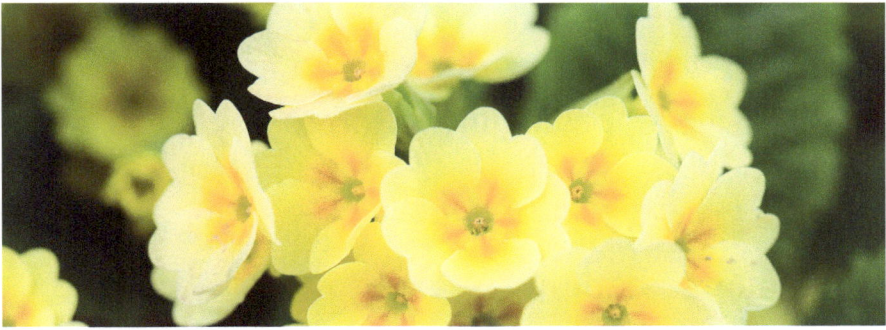

Primrose Night Treatment

This is a beautiful serum that promotes anti-aging, reduces lines and wrinkles and balances hormones.

Ingredients:

- 1 teaspoon of evening primrose oil
- 2 drops of geranium essential oil
- 1 drop lavender essential oil
- 1 capsule of vitamin E oil

How To

1. Mix evening primrose oil, geranium and lavender oil into a small amber glass bottle.
2. Pour 1 capsule of Vitamin E into the mixture.
3. Gently shake to mix.

4. In the evening after cleansing, apply the blend to your face, paying attention to any areas of redness and wrinkles.
5. Let it soak in for at least 10 minutes before heading to bed.

Its Power!

Geranium oil is an astringent, it induces contractions deep within the skin. It has the power to minimize wrinkles, as it tightens and slows down the effects of aging.

Evening primrose rectifies hormonal acne, heals scars and sun damage. It prevents and reverses age-related changes in skin tissue.

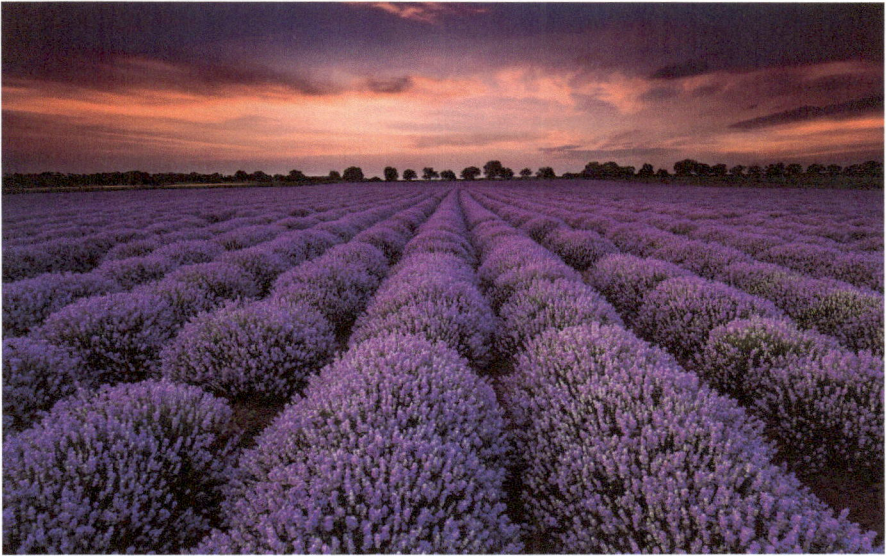

Lavender Dream

Lavender Dream is a luxurious body and face lotion. The aroma will linger all day, providing you with nutrients of the body and mind.

Ingredients:
- 1/2 cup jojoba oil
- 1/4 cup coconut oil
- 1/4 cup raw beeswax
- 1 teaspoon vitamin E oil
- 2 tablespoon shea butter
- 10 drops lavender essential oil
- 3 drops frankincense essential oil

How to

1. Combine jojoba, coconut, beeswax oil in a double boiler or a glass bowl sitting in a saucepan.
2. Stir as the oils melt.
3. Add shea butter and mix to combined.
4. Remove front heat.
5. Add vitamin E oil and all essential oils.
6. Pour into a small/medium glass jar with a shallow base.
7. A little goes a long way.
8. Best if used within 5 months.

Its Power!

Excellent for Anti-aging, damaged and dry skin, sunburns, diaper rash, stretch marks or eczema. Can be used on face or body. Soothing and ultra-hydrating. The oil combinations are deep penetrating.

Lavender is proven to improves cellular communication, and helps your body produce three of the most powerful antioxidants: glutathione, catalase and superoxide dismutase.

While the frankincense protects skin cells, reduces blemishes, pores, prevent wrinkles, and lifts and tighten skin.

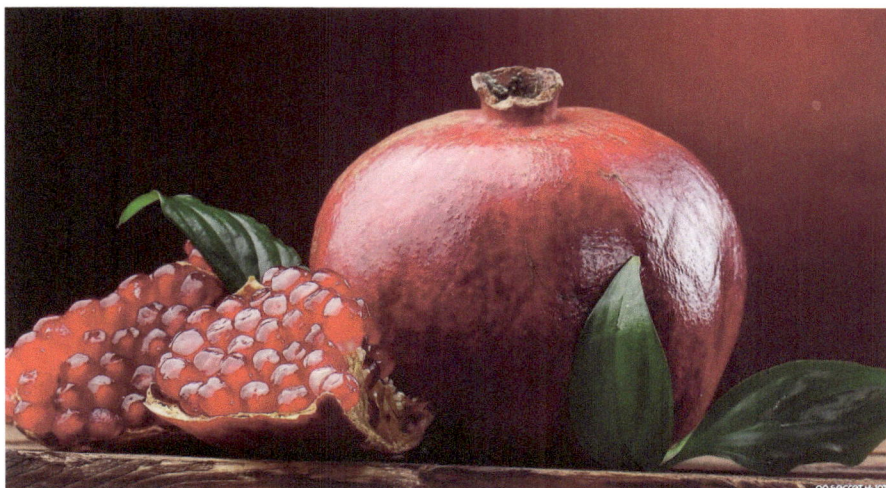

Coconut Pom Young Butter

The coconut and pomegranate combination will be your new favorite skin glowing butter. Slather the rich butter across your entire body, and experience a brighter day. This simple recipe offers a plethora of skin loving nutrients and protection from the sun.

Ingredients:
- 1 cup coconut oil
- 1 tsp. vitamin E oil
- 1 tsp. pomegranate seed oil

How to

1. **Do not melt the coconut oil first.** It will only whip up if it's solid.
2. Put all ingredients into a mixing bowl.
3. Mix on high speed with a wire whisk for 5-8 minutes or until whipped into a light, airy consistency.
4. Spoon the whipped butter into a glass jar.
5. Store at room temperature, or in the refrigerator.
6. Your skin butter should stay soft, even at colder temperatures.

Its Power!

Pomegranate seed oil stimulates major cells found in the outer layer of the skin. This helps to reverse skin damage, rejuvenates skin and creates a youthful appearance.

The dark color of the seed oil also protects your skin from sun damage. It contains an SPF, and can be used as a natural sunblock and sunscreen.

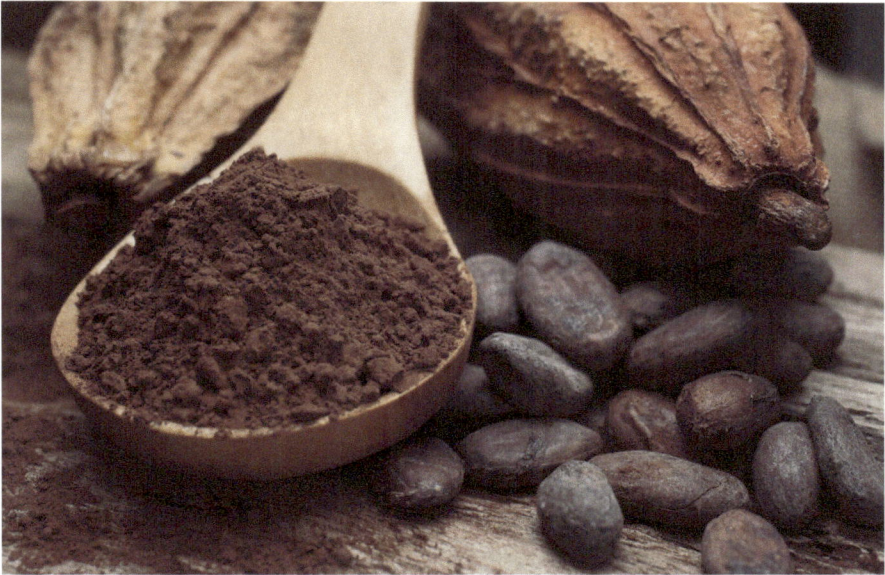

Chocolate-Mint Hydrating Butter

Dazzle in this chocolate mint hydrating butter. You will look and feel as good as you smell. This butter is loaded with a natural pain reliever and stress reducer, along with fats that bring youth back to your skin.

Ingredients:
- 1/2 cup cocoa butter
- 1/2 cup coconut oil
- 30-40 drops peppermint essential oil

How To

1. Add chilled coconut oil and cocoa butter to your mixing bowl.
2. Add peppermint essential oil.
3. Turn on the mixer slow at first.
4. Speed up as the oils begin incorporating (medium-high speed).
5. Scrape the mixing bowl every few minutes to distribute evenly.
6. Mix for a total of 8 minutes or until your butter is perfectly whipped and airy.
7. Scoop your chocolate-mint whipped hydrating butter into a glass jar.
8. Apply as needed on entire body.

Its Power!

Coco butter is loaded with saturated fats that are especially beneficial for healing dry, cracked skin, improve elasticity and tone, better collagen retention and production, and supercharges skin hydration.

Peppermint is an ancient oil used for its natural pain relief. It is a very effective natural painkiller and muscle relaxant. It is especially helpful in soothing an aching back, sore muscles, and melting away a tension headache. Peppermint aids in healing wounds, sunburns, acne and other skin irritations. It also reduces allergens to pollen and acts as a decongestant.

This beautiful recipe provides you with a long lasting natural bug repellent. Bugs hate peppermint!

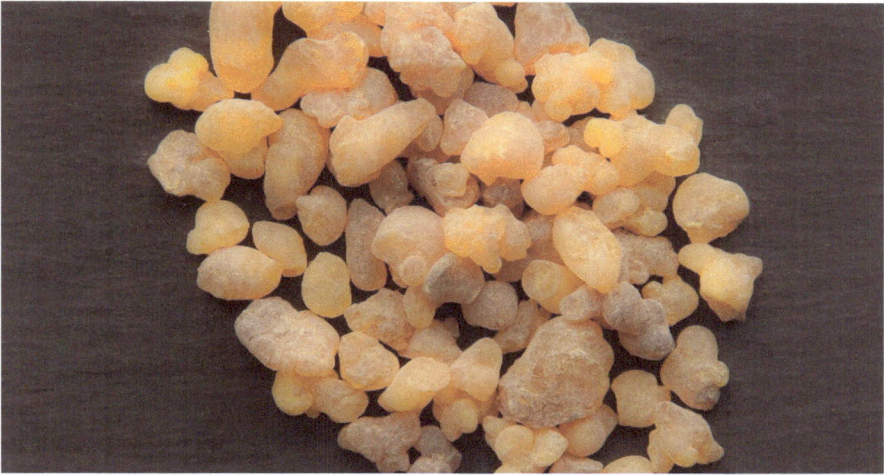

Whipped Frankincense Cream

This is an amazing Frankincense day and night cream for your face and neck. This is the kind of cream that sells out before it even hits the shelf. Its glorious in every way!

Ingredients:

- 1 cup cocoa butter
- 1/4 cup coconut oil
- 2 Tbsp. jojoba oil
- 2 Tbsp. sweet almond oil
- 35 drops frankincense essential oil

How To

1. Bring cocoa butter to room temperature or slightly soft.
2. Combine softened cocoa butter, coconut oil, jojoba oil, and almond oil in a mixing bowl.
3. Place the bowl into your fridge until it starts to harden.
4. Then whip the oils with a mixer until you achieve an airy consistently.
5. Slowly add frankincense until mixed well.
6. Use small amount on your neck and face day and night.
7. Keep in a cool place in a glass container.

Its Power!

Frankincense essential oil is a powerful astringent, it is superior at protecting skin cells. It naturally slows signs of aging, dramatically reduces wrinkles and tightens skin. The oil can be used anywhere where the skin becomes saggy, such as the abdomen, jaw or around eyes.

Frankincense has been considered the most luxurious oil for thousands of years. It has been used by royalty since the beginning of its discovery in ancient times.

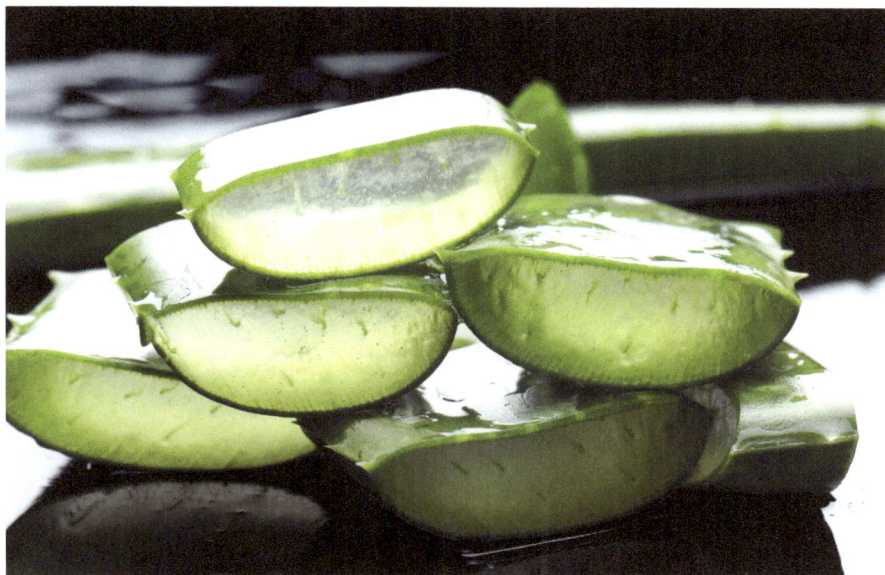

Soothing Aloe Body & Face Cream

The Soothing Aloe Cream is an aphrodisiac. It not only melts your entire body into a deep relaxation, but it also induces sensuality for both male and female.

Ingredients:

- 1/8 cup aloe vera gel
- 1/8 cup coconut oil softened (not melted)
- 1 vitamin E capsule or 1/2 tsp vitamin E oil
- 5 drops frankincense essential oil
- 5-10 drops ylang ylang essential oil

How To

1. Whisk together the aloe vera gel, coconut oil and vitamin E oil.
2. Add the essential oils.
3. Mix well.
4. Use for entire body and face.
5. Store in a cool dry place.
6. Excellent for sunburns, after showers or shaving.

Its Power!

Frankincense reduces the appearance of scars and stretch marks. it is a great astringent for face and body acne, antibacterial, tightens skin and reduced wrinkles.

Aloe vera accelerates wound healing, reduce acne and infection, and dramatically lightens blemishes. It is rich in vitamins C and E and beta carotene. Aloe vera contains anti-inflammatory and antimicrobial properties, taking years off your face and body.

Ylang Ylang when applied to the skin preserves a "youthful glow" and help prevent signs of aging. It is even powerful at fighting the development of skin cancer cells and melanoma. Ylang ylang is also a natural aphrodisiac.

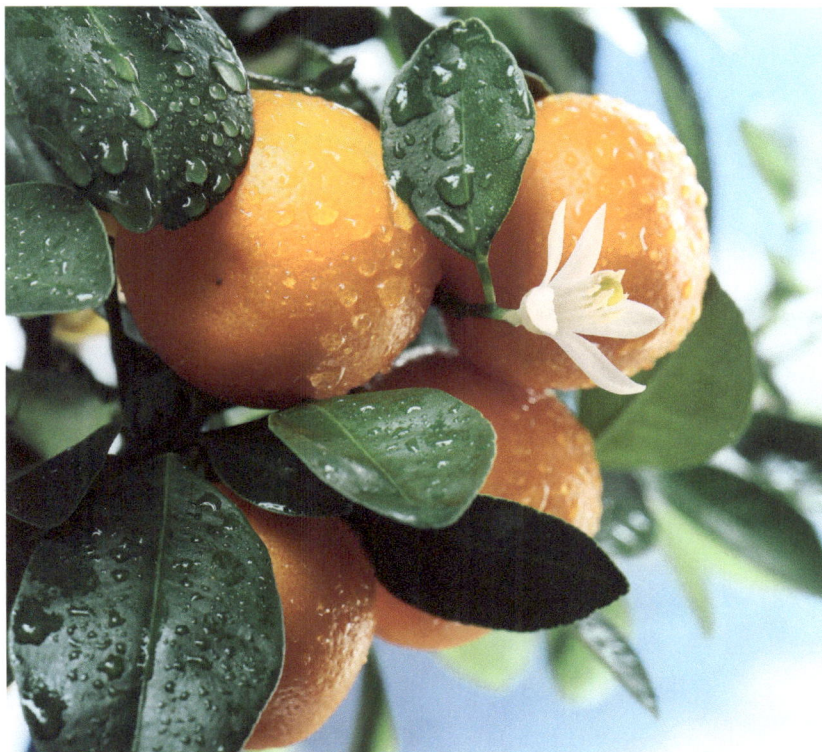

Orange Rejuvenation

If you are suffering from dark spots, deep wrinkles, and poor skin quality; this ultra-hydrating cream is for you. If you want to defy your age, then the concentration of vitamin C and the pomegranates cellular deliver system will get you there.

Ingredients:
- ¼ cup coconut oil
- 10 drops orange essential oil
- 11 drops lavender essential oil

- 1 tsp. pomegranate seed oil
- 10 drops ylang-ylang essential oil

How To

1. Add coconut oil and all essential oils together.
2. Mix well.
3. Pour into a small glass container.
4. Use as needed (a little goes a long ways).
5. Citrus oils can cause the skin to become more sensitive to the sun.

Its Power!

Orange oil is known to provide extremely high levels of vitamin C that protects, heals, and fights sign of aging. It also removes dark spots, increases collagen production, boost circulation and protects the skin against some cancers. Orange also destroys bacteria and inflammation that is known to cause acne.

Pomegranate seed oil helps channel nutrients directly to the cell, accelerating cellular regeneration and rejuvenation of the skin. It is anti-carcinogenic, and supports immune, hormonal, circulatory, and metabolic health in male and female.

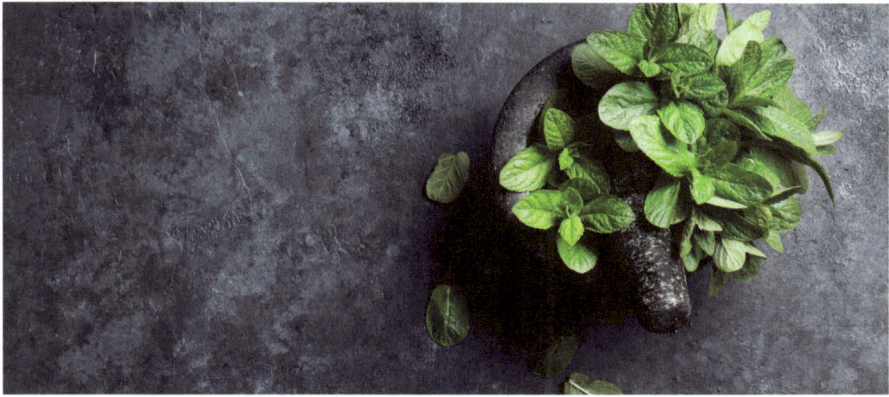

Peppermint Skin Salve

The peppermint skin salve is soothing and relieves pain associated with arthritis or skin injury. Next time you are having back, knee, feet or wrist pain from being overworked, rub a small amount on the affected area and enjoy the relaxation. This salve is excellent to have on hand for most small injuries or general soreness.

Ingredient:
- ¼ cup shea butter
- ¼ cup coconut oil
- 3 Tbsp. beeswax
- ¼ cup magnesium flakes and 2 Tbsp. boiling water
- 10 drops oregano essential oil
- 10 drops peppermint essential oil

How To

1. Pour 2 tablespoons of boiling water in to the magnesium flakes and stir until it dissolves.
2. Let this thick mixture cool.
3. Combine coconut oil, beeswax and shea butter into a double broiler and turn on low heat. You can also put 1 inch of water in a saucepan and sit a glass jar inside.
4. When melted, let it cool to room temperature and slightly opaque.
5. If in a bowl, use a hand blender or immersion blender on medium speed and start blending the oil mixture.
6. Slowly add the magnesium mixture and continue to blend.
7. Add the essential oils and continue to blend.
8. Put in the fridge for 15-45 minutes.
9. Once the salve begins to harden re-blend to get body butter consistency. Store in fridge for a cooling lotion or at room temp for up to two months.

Its Power!

When oregano essential oil is applied topically, it reduces redness and skin irritation. It also relieves pain that is associated with arthritis or injury to the skin. Oregano oil provides superior protection against bacterial and fungal infections.

Magnesium is present in every organ in our body. It's a vital mineral for 300 reactions that regulate our health. It is known to reduce stress-related skin irritations and speed up healing time.

Peppermint is an ancient remedy used for its anti-microbial, anti-fungal, and anti-parasitic qualities. It is used to treat bacterial, fungal, and parasitic infections, both internally and externally.

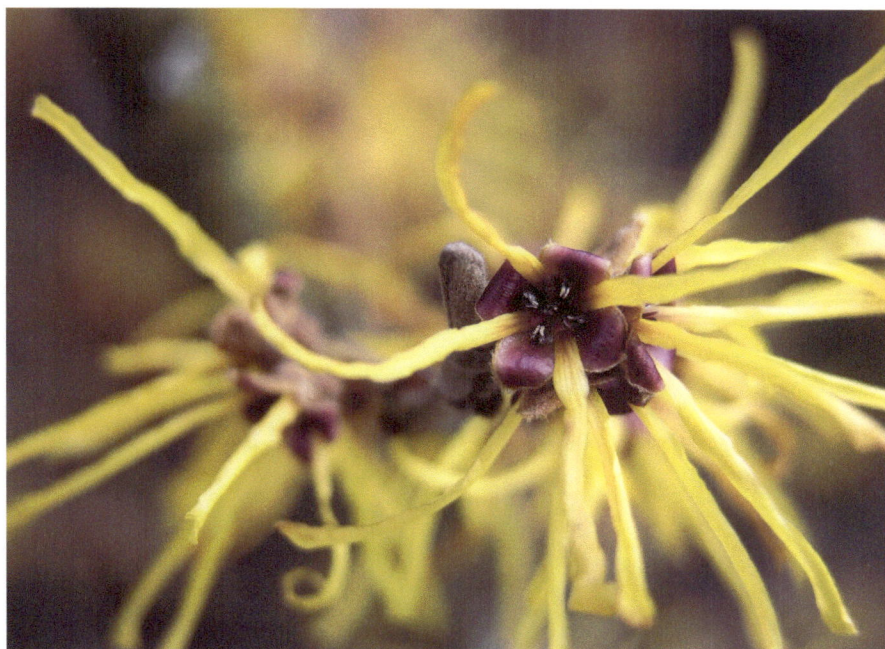

Witches Tree Skin Toner

This is a magical 2-ingredient toner that removes makeup residue and tighten your pores. Even when you thought your skin was completely clean, this toner will pull gunk out from everywhere. Once you try this toner, you will never feel clean without it.

Ingredients:
- 2 drops of tea tree essential oil
- 1 oz. witch hazel

How To

1. Add tea tree oil and witch hazel in a small glass jar.
2. Shake it up.
3. Then saturate a cotton pad and gently wipe your face using an upward motion from jawline to forehead (avoiding your eyes).

Its Power!

Tea tree oil can quickly clear up the sebum glands and eliminate the bacteria, resulting in smoother, healthier-looking skin.

Witch hazel is excellent for acne-prone skin. It reduces the look of pores, stops excess oil production, and it helps prevent the development of whiteheads and blackheads. It also contains a high level of polyphenols, the same compounds used to create supplements that slow down disease and premature aging.

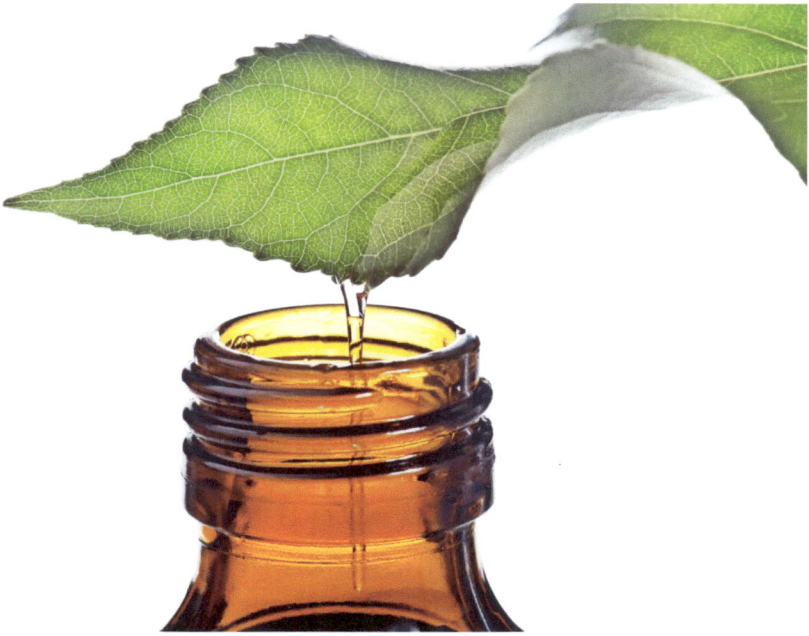

Tea Tree Blemish Paste

This is a miracle worker for deep cystic acne, whitehead and blackheads.

Ingredients:

- 1 ½ tsp. pure baking soda
- 1 tsp. purified water
- 1 drop tea tree essential oil

How To

1. Combine water, baking soda and mix to a creamy paste.
2. Add tea tree oil.

3. Apply the paste on the acne affected areas.
4. Let paste sit on your face for 2-10 minutes.
5. Rinse paste off thoroughly with warm water.
6. Repeat the process 1x per week.

Its Power!

Tea tree essential oil kills Propionibacterium acnes that live inside hair follicles and can lead to inflammation. The oil also contains soothing properties that help calm the burning and itching of flare-ups.

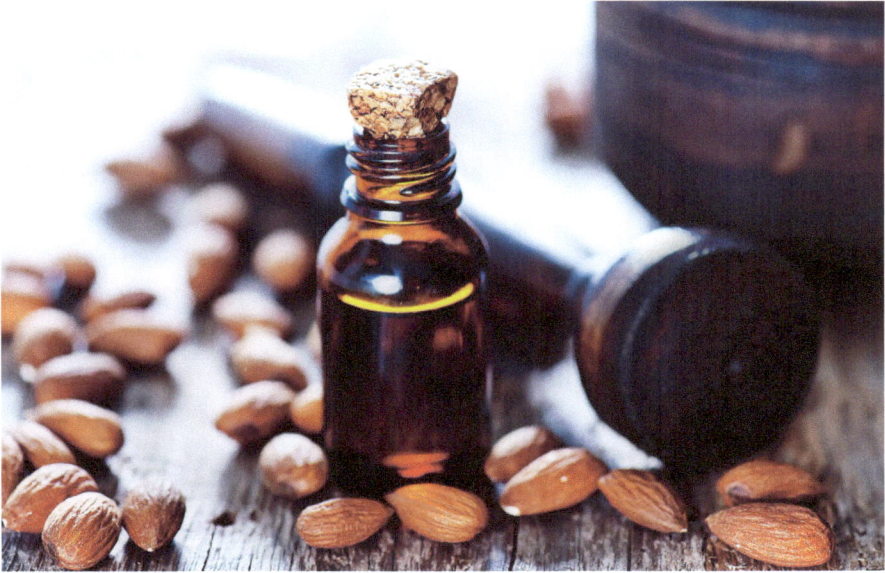

Sweet Almond Shaving Cream

The Sweet Almond Shaving Cream feels as good as it sounds. Its nutrient rich properties penetrate deep to remove ingrown hairs and rashes before they even start. The aroma of the sweet almond and coconut is uplifting. Add lavender essential oil for a more feminine aroma.

Ingredients:
- 4 Tbsp. solid shea butter
- 3 Tbsp. coconut oil
- 2 Tbsp. sweet almond oil
- 10 drops of lavender (optional)

How To

1. Using a double boiler, (or a glass bowl inside a saucepan of warm water) add the shea butter and coconut oil.
2. Remove from heat once completely melted.
3. Add almond EO or lavender for a more feminine aroma (EO is optional).
4. Stir well.
5. Transfer bowl to the fridge and let the mixture harden.
6. Use a mixer to whip until it is the consistency of frosting.
7. Let it sit 20 minutes before transferring to an airtight container.

Its Power!

Sweet almond oil is a mild, hypoallergenic oil that can be safely used even on the most sensitive skin.

Almond oil is light in texture, and can easily penetrate deep into the skin, softening and removing dirt and debris accumulated in the skin pores and hair follicles. This prevents blackheads, acne, ingrown hair and more. Thanks to the Vitamin A content, it reduces redness and irritation.

Sweet almond oil is rich in Vitamin E, monounsaturated fatty acids, proteins, potassium and zinc. It is optimal skin food.

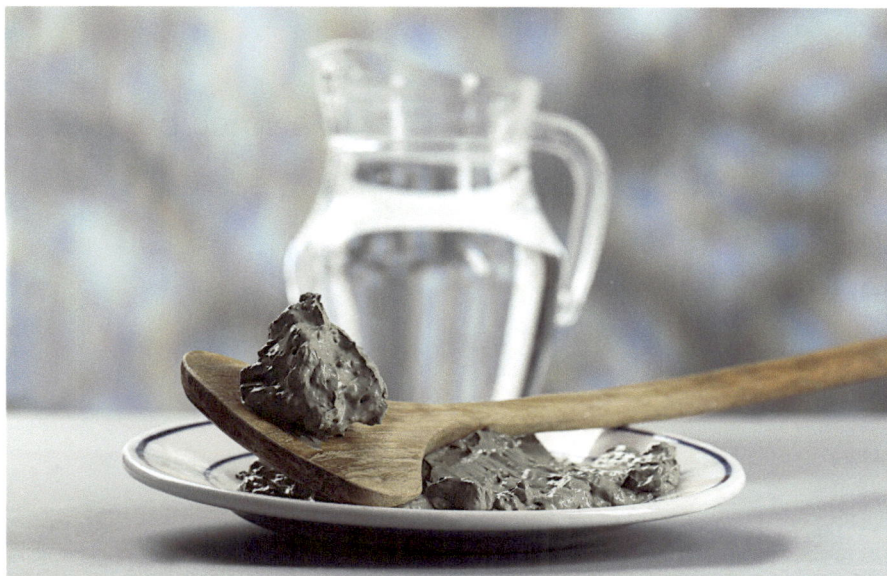

Bentonite Clay Detox Mask

The bentonite clay detox mask is essential to luxurious skin. No skin care routine is complete without a mask that removes all the grime, dead skin, bacteria and toxins left in the pores.

Ingredients:

- 2 Tbsp. bentonite clay
- 1 Tsp. coconut oil
- ½ Tbsp. raw honey
- 1 drop of lemon essential oil

How To

1. Mix all ingredients together in a small bowl.
2. apply to a freshly washed face.
3. Let the mask sit for 10 minutes.
4. Rinse well.
5. Use as desired or 1-4 times per month.

Its Power!

When bentonite clay is left to dry on the skin, it binds to bacteria and toxins within pores and completely extract them. Its special ability to act as an antibiotic treatment when applied topically to the skin, can also eliminate skin infections and speed up healing time of wounds.

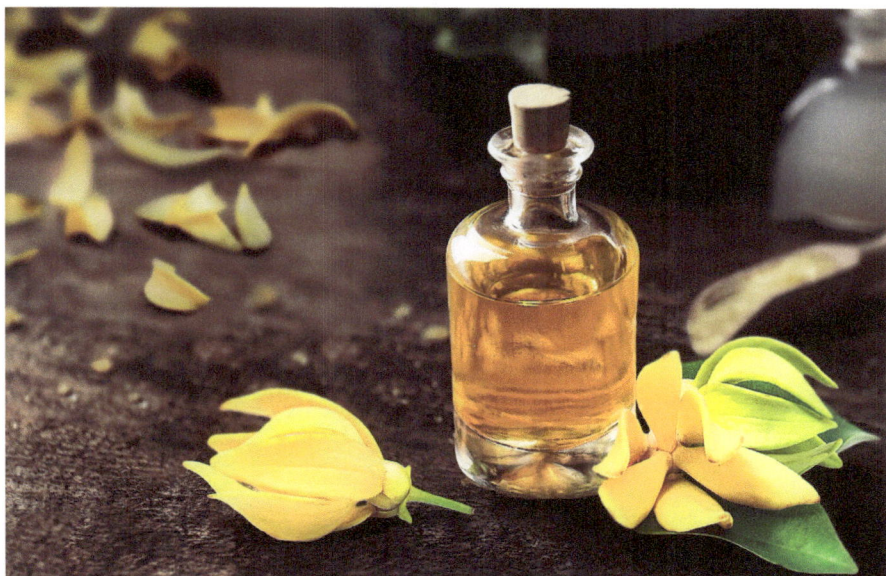

Ylang Ylang Foaming Face Wash

This foaming face wash will send you to the moon with its incredible aroma. Ylang ylang is an aphrodisiac along with patchouli. The lemon grass and sweet almond oils tantalize your senses, while providing a first-class deep cleansing experience.

Ingredients:

- 1/2 tsp sweet almond oil
- 1/3 cup castile soap
- 10 drops ylang ylang essential oil
- 6 drops patchouli essential oil
- 4 drops lemongrass essential oil
- 2/3 cup filtered water

How To

1. Pour the castile soap, and sweet almond oil into a foaming soap dispenser.
2. Add the essential oils and swirl to combine.
3. Fill the container with filtered water and screw on.
4. Give a light swirl or shake before each use.
5. Use daily.

Its Power!

Ylang ylang It is extremely effective at maintaining moisture and oil balance of the skin. It keeps the skin looking hydrated, smooth, and young.

Patchouli oil has the power to stimulate hormones and increase your sex drive. It stimulates muscle contractions tightening sagging skin. Patchouli regenerates new skin cells and is great for all skin types. When used at night it reduces the symptoms of insomnia.

Lemongrass is a powerful cleanser. it's an antiseptic and astringent, sterilizes your pores, serve as a natural toner, and strengthen your skin tissues. Lemongrass also eases headaches associated with stress and tension.

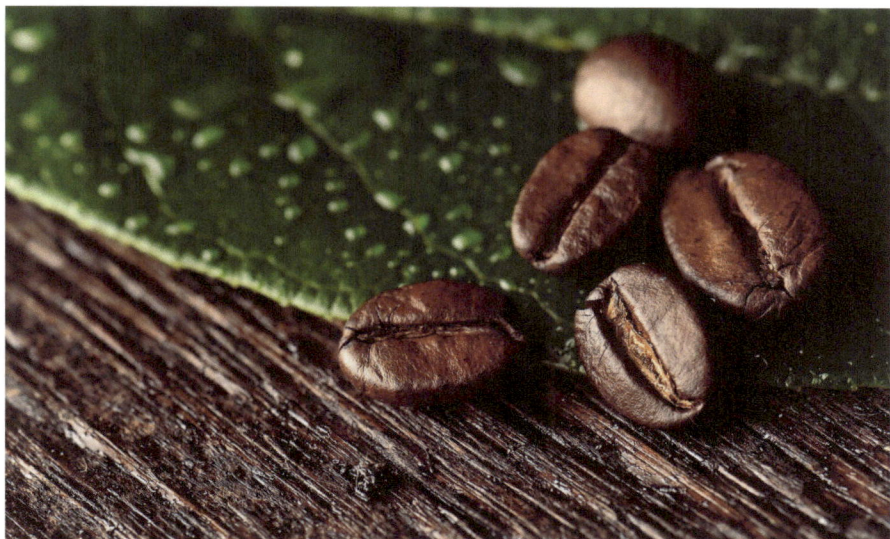

Coffee-Coconut Body Scrub

This scrub will not let you down. It is a simple yet brilliant combination of skin loving oil, and a nutrient rich/caffeinated exfoliant. Your entire body will glow for days.

Ingredients:

- ½ tsp. coconut oil
- ½ tsp. finely ground coffee beans

How To

1. Mix together the coconut oil and ground coffee.
2. Apply to your face or body using circular motions.

3. Leave on for at least 15 minutes or up to an hour.
4. Rinse off with warm water.
5. Use 2-3 times per week.

Its Power!

Coffee is a rich source of antioxidants that protects our skin against free radicals. The caffeine in coffee stimulates skin and improves blood flow and increases the production of collagen and elastin.

It also minimizes fine lines and protects against the loss of moisture. Coffee helps reverse the damage of UV rays!

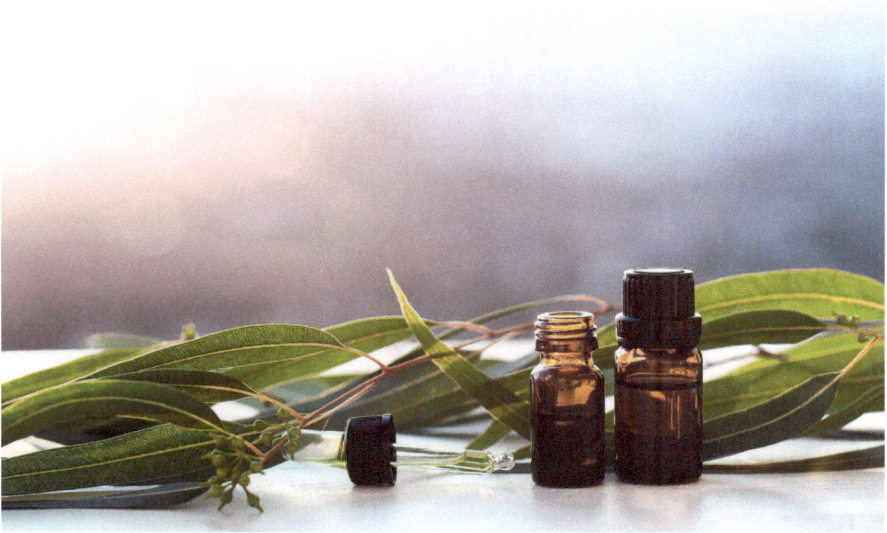

Eucalyptus Sunscreen Bar

There is nothing better than rubbing your entire body with a natural sunscreen that smells like paradise.

Ingredients:
- 1/2 cup shea butter
- 5 Tbsp. beeswax
- 1/2 cup coconut oil
- 2 Tbsp. zinc oxide (see SPF chart below)
- ½ tsp vitamin E oil
- 20-30 drops eucalyptus essential oil

How To

1. Combine the shea butter, coconut oil and beeswax in a glass bowl placed over a warm pot of water or use a double boiler.
2. Heat on low until the ingredients are melted and fully incorporated.
3. Remove from heat and stir in the zinc oxide, the essential oil, and the vitamin E oil.
4. Pour into silicone molds and place in the fridge to cool for about 30-60 minutes.
5. Pop out and store in an airtight container.
6. Store at room temperature.
7. These homemade sunscreen lotion bars will melt in the hot sun. keep in airtight container – in a cooler when out on hot days. When you go back indoors it will solidify again if left out in the sun.
8. You simply rub all over your body while holding the bar in your hand. You can rub it in further with your hands.

FOR SUNSCREEN SPF GRADES:

- For SPF 2-5 Use 5% zinc oxide
- For SPF 6-11 Use 10% zinc oxide
- For SPF 12-19 Use 15% zinc oxide
- For SPF 20+ Use 20% zinc oxide

Its Power!

Eucalyptus oil gives you soft to the touch, blemish-free skin. It even cools your body down as the outside heat rises. Eucalyptus is a wonderful skin healing oil.